LIPEDEMA DIET FOR WOMEN

A Beginner's 3-Week Step-by-Step Guide,
With Sample Recipes and a Meal Plan

Mary Golanna

mindplusfood

DISCLAIMER

By reading this disclaimer, you are accepting the terms of the disclaimer in full. If you disagree with this disclaimer, please do not read the guide.

All of the content within this guide is provided for informational and educational purposes only, and should not be accepted as independent medical or other professional advice. The author is not a doctor, physician, nurse, mental health provider, or registered nutritionist/dietician. Therefore, using and reading this guide does not establish any form of a physician-patient relationship.

Always consult with a physician or another qualified health provider with any issues or questions you might have regarding any sort of medical condition. Do not ever disregard any qualified professional medical advice or delay seeking that advice because of anything you have read in this guide. The information in this guide is not intended to be any sort of medical advice and should not be used in lieu of any medical advice by a licensed and qualified medical professional.

The information in this guide has been compiled from a variety of known sources. However, the author cannot attest to or guarantee the accuracy of each source and thus should not be held liable for any errors or omissions.

You acknowledge that the publisher of this guide will not be held

CONTENTS

INTRODUCTION

Did you know that approximately 1 out of every 9 adult females are diagnosed with lipedema worldwide?

Lipedema is a chronic disease in which the fatty tissue under the skin starts accumulating abnormally. It is also called lipoedema or lipodema. Women are more often affected than men, and it appears almost always after puberty. Typically, the feet and legs are most severely affected at first, but over time the disease can progress to include the hips, buttocks and upper limbs. In later stages it may also affect other parts of the body such as the abdomen, breasts and hands.

In women with lipedema, fat tissue accumulates at a rate that is much lower than normal after puberty, but not as low as in obesity. The affected areas become enlarged and the skin of the affected parts of the body distends, becoming smooth and dimpled. These changes resemble those of normal pregnancy

Lipedema must neither be confused with obesity nor with lymphedema. In obesity, fat accumulates in the whole body, and in lymphedema accumulation and swelling occur on one side of the body. While in the case of lipedema fat occurs in the limbs, sparing the hands and feet.

It is also not edema but a related adipose tissue disorder also known as Adiposis Dolorosa. It is important to spread awareness, conduct research, and identify better diagnostic and treatment methods for lipedema so the affected women can obtain the care that they need and deserve.

If you want to get more information about the disorder, how it is diagnosed, its treatments, and cures, eating habits and relation to this particular condition, continue reading.

In this guide, you will come to discover...
- What lipedema is
- Differences between lipedema, obesity, edema, and lymphedema
- Treatment and medication for lipedema
- Foods to eat and avoid if you have lipedema
- A 3-week diet plan with sample recipes

LIPEDEMA – COMMON ADIPOSE TISSUE DISORDER

In a very simple and understandable way, Lipedema means "fluid in the fat." It is known to be a painful fat disorder. In Lipedema, fat gets deposited on the legs, thighs, buttocks, and upper arm in a bilateral and sometimes in a symmetrical manner.

Initially described by Allen and Hines in 1940, it was little understood, misdiagnosed, mistreated, and got confused with lymphedema and obesity. Till now the dilemma of misdiagnosis persists and many women have to suffer because the disease is typically dismissed simply as obesity.

Lipedema might begin at the onset of puberty, during pregnancy, or at the time of menopause due to hormonal changes. The exact cause of this painful fat syndrome is still unknown but according to some researchers it might be a hereditary disease and a particular gene could be responsible for it.

Symptoms
Below is a list of symptoms associated with Lipedema. In case of delayed diagnosis, symptoms may worsen:
● Disproportionate accumulation of fat on legs and hips compared

to the upper body
- Symmetrical swelling on both sides of the body is affected equally.
- Does not affect hands and feet
- Knee joint appears to be covered with fat and have loose and floppy connective tissues
- Fat that looks like cellulite and feels soft
- Tenderness and bruising to affected areas
- Affected areas may become pale and cold

Differentiating Lymphedema and Edema
Many doctors misdiagnosed lipedema as edema but it is one of the severe forms of edema. In medical terms, edema means swelling, and in the case of Lipedema, swelling of fat-storing cells occurs. These cells (adipocytes) are present under the skin.

Compared to Lymphedema, Lipedema is associated with serious pain and palpation. Lymphedema is a lymphatic system disorder and is commonly caused by dysfunction in the flow of lymph fluid through the arms or legs. It also affects the hands and feet.

Stages of lipedema
Lipedema consists of 5 major types, from which 1 to 3 are most common.

Stage 1: Involves a smooth and even skin surface with a buildup of hypodermis but nodules could be felt.
Stage 2: Skin becomes uneven and a nodular or mass-like appearance of fat appears on the skin. Connective tissues also got thickened.
Stage 3: Involves large growths of fat mass that cause deformation of the thighs and area around the knee.
Stage 4: Involves the presence of lipo-lymphedema. It occurs when lipedema is associated with lymphedema,

Treatment and management

Unfortunately, no cure is present to treat Lipedema but there are certain things that could prevent its prevalence and stop it from becoming worse.

Your lifestyle can help it from getting worse.

● Diet
Healthy eating slows down the progression of the disease by maintaining a healthy weight. A recent study revealed that adapting a Ketogenic diet could reduce the progression of the disease.

● Exercise
Exercises including swimming, riding a bicycle, and walking help you to maintain your mobility. Swimming will mobilize the fluid and soften the tissues while biking will help calf and foot muscles to get relaxed.

● Use of Stockings and Bandages
Compression stockings and bandages help you to reduce pain and feeling of discomfort, also help you in easy walking.

Besides these, other treatments of Lipedema may include a form of conservative treatment. Before going towards a complex treatment, first, try this. Gentle massage and certain types of skin stretching along with wrapping techniques help reduce pain and inflammation.

● Liposuction
When conservative treatments fail to control Lipedema, "liposuction" is suggested by most doctors. During liposuction, excessive fat is removed in a way that lymphatic vessels may not get damaged. The water-jet-assisted liposuction (WAL) technique is commonly used. Klein solution or saline is used as a jet that releases the fat for liposuction. No waiting period is required to tumescent the tissue after anesthesia. Furthermore, the tumescent technique and Laser-assisted liposuction techniques

are also used. Although liposuction is a costly treatment it reduces pain, muscle cramps, and bruising by reading the fat content and helps improve your mobility.

In addition to these treatments, appropriate education of the disease, motivational and inspirational movements, counseling to focus on healthy eating, and social interactions will have positive outcomes. These steps of awareness and motivation are necessary because individuals suffering from lipedema may get depression and anxiety issues.

LIPEDEMA AND WOMEN

As discussed earlier, lipedema is affecting 1 of every 9 women in the USA, and onset are typically associated with puberty, pregnancy, or menopause.

Women with lipedema are overweight and they are thought to be obese, which is an injustice to them. Early diagnosis and treatment surely stop or slow down the progression of the disease. But if left untreated or mistreated, it could be chronic. Females have a much heavier lower body than the upper part and fat continues to accumulate from below the abdomen to downward.

A sad fact about the patients with lipedema is that the patients tend to gain weight in the lipidemic areas and can only lose it in the non-lipidemic areas. That's a serious element of concern for those women who tried weight loss treatments to get rid of lipedema. Because such treatments will have effects only on non-lipedema or areas above the waistline.

Lipedema concerns the women's health and quality of life of females and their daily routine is badly affected due to this disorder which has no geographical boundaries and impacts about 11-15% of women worldwide. Ladies are more conscious about their beauty and physique but uneven body shape due to concentrated fat in the lower body proves to be a somewhat inferiority complex for them.

In an article "Women's Experiences of Living with Lipedema" published in "Healthcare for Women International," women were interviewed to know what they felt and what others judge about them. According to them, women with lipedema are body-shamed in public and also they get no serious attention from doctors. Furthermore, there are also other analyses done by researchers which are summarized below.

Dominated by erratic and weighty body
Taking even a single step is hard for lipedema women, hence, feeling their bodies a burden. Moving around with large, uneven, bulky legs is a painful and harsh activity for them. Such women are unable to perform daily-life activities because other organs are under the pressure of their giant bodies and legs. This pressure is from both inside and outside, mental and physical. They feel like the blood vessels and nerves will explode, and this continuous pain becomes a nightmare for them.

One of the interviewed women expressed the pain and said it's like someone is pricking you. She could not meet anyone and had to rest all the time.

Lipedemic women felt their burdensome body as unattractive for their spouses and this uneven and bumpy feeling could be challenging for their sexual life too. The folds and bumps in the big fatty body might be home to infections, itching, smell, etc. which could be a hindrance to closeness to their partners.

Not supported by healthcare professionals
When lipidemic women start feeling unusual changes in their body they consult a healthcare professional. After a long process of examinations, when the doctors are unable to exactly diagnose the issue, they recommend weight-loss exercises and a healthy diet. Sometimes such women often confront pessimism and have to face harsh comments from their doctors.

Healthcare professionals don't listen to their patients who want to say that certain medicines are not acting on them. They use to touch them in a reckless way and awkwardly question them, hurting patients' self-respect and dignity. The doctors don't want to show their lack of knowledge but there are few who open up upon this. One of the ladies described that she was lucky to have such a good doctor.

On the contrary, if the woman, by chance gets diagnosed (because diagnosis is difficult due to lack of knowledge about lipedema), the next step is even more difficult. She felt alone in making the decision about her treatment, to whom would she discuss the situation? And to whom she consults for financial support? Because people again think that she is simply obese and needs to change her lifestyle.

During interviews, women described that they are treated in different ways. Upon diagnosis, few are recommended to use compression garments and others are told to have lymph massages. Women also undergo surgeries like gastric surgery or liposuction.

Body-shamed due to bulky appearance
Women complained that they are not being understood by the people around them and were bantered for being overweight. This is really painful when someone is struggling with lipedema and people called him obese and fatty. People without knowing the pain and sorrow of lipidemic females, gaze at him and stare at him in a disgusting manner.

"My God, what big legs she has"
"Those legs do not fit your body"
"Fat one" or "the one with the big legs
"What happened to you? You looked so nice last year."

These comments really hurt the women in illness.

Unable to take responsibility and feeling guilt

Women suffering from lipedema are unable to participate in daily life activities. On the other side when they fail to manage themselves and fail to handle their illness they start blaming themselves. They feel guilty for being a burden to the family and relatives. Sometimes when the woman does not even help the family in routine activities and support her spouse financially, she feels herself a burden on her husband.

Lipidemic women felt bad when they could not take care of their children, they could not cuddle or allow their kids to sit in their laps. Eating unhealthy at certain rare events, eating less, exercising, everything seems of no use because starvation and exercise have nothing to do with lipedema. If eating unhealthy, other peoples' compliments would be painful. An interviewed woman described that strong willpower is the only factor that could help fight against lipedema.

Women need moral and physical support from others but are left alone in many cases. To help women facing lipedema, patients' social media groups and associations are created. Women in such groups feel a sense of ease that they don't have to express their pain. These groups create a sense of companionship among women where their pain could be understood without explaining.

MANAGING LIPEDEMA WITH DIET AND NUTRITION

L ipedema is a common adipose tissue disorder in women which is often misdiagnosed and confused with obesity. As we have discussed earlier, there is no particular cure for this disease but still, slight changes to lifestyle would have positive impacts. We all know that a healthy and balanced diet is a guarantee of good health.

Many healthcare professionals, who diagnose lipedema and strive to find the best treatments, also recommend the addition and elimination of certain food items from the diet according to the body's conditions. Some even say that the Paleo Diet is a good option.

Having the right diet may not directly cure the disease but help in reducing the symptoms like inflammation, bruising, pain, swelling, etc., and a fat-free diet will obviously have positive effects.

Keeping in view the severity of fat-related disorders Dr. Karen Herbst, an endocrinologist from the University of California, based in the USA, has developed the Rare Adipose Disorder Diet

(RAD Diet). People and women, in particular, who are suffering from lipedema, should opt for a RAD diet to reduce inflammation in their bodies.

Below is a detailed description of the principles of the RAD diet, which could help you to choose what to eat and what to avoid.

Foods you should eat	Eat in limited amount	Eat rarely or Avoid these foods
PROTEINS		
White and Oily Fish Organic Free Range Eggs	Free Range Chicken Seafood	Processed Meat, Bacon, Ham, Salami, Sausages, Grain Fed Meat, Mass Reared Chicken, Factory Farmed Eggs, Wheat Protein.
FRUITS		
Berries, Citrus Fruits, Banana, Cherries, Avocado, Olives	Melon, Kiwi, Grapes, Pineapple, Mango, Apple, Pears, Plums, Peaches, Apricots	Canned fruit, Dried Fruit
VEGETABLES		
Green Vegetables, Colorful Vegetables,	Sweet Potatoes	Potatoes in all forms, Corn, Canned Vegetables

Squashes, Onions, Garlic, Mushrooms, Herbs		
NUTS AND SEEDS		
Unsalted Tree Nuts and Seeds, Brazil Nuts		Roasted and Salted Nuts, Peanuts
GRAINS AND CARBS		
Whole grains like brown rice, quinoa, feta	White flour, white rice, white potatoes, Chickpea, Buckwheat, millet	Ready to eat or processed cereals, ray products (like pizza, bread, biscuits, cakes)
FATS AND OILS		
Extra-Virgin Olive Oil, Nut Oils, Avocado Oil, Coconut Oil, Cocoa Butter, Flaxseed Oil, Sesame Seeds Oil	Hydrogenated oils- but prefer not to eat	Margarines, Hydrogenated Fats, Partially Hydrogenated Fats, Vegetable Oils e.g. (Sunflower, Rapeseed, Corn, Mixed Palm) Fried Foods e.g. (chips, crisps)
DAIRY PRODUCTS		
Organic Butter or Ghee, Goat's Milk, Cheese From Goats and Sheep	Organic Grass Fed Cow's Milk Cheese	Low-Fat Plain and Flavored Yogurts, Evaporated Milk, Condensed Milk, Ice Cream

OTHERS		
Green Tea, Herb And Fruit tea, Naturally Decaffeinated Coffee And Tea Coconut Milk, Fresh and Dried Spices, Fresh and Dried Herbs, Fermented Foods, Non-Sugary Condiments	Home-Made Smoothies, Caffeinated, Coffee and Tea, White Spirits, Red Wine Dark chocolate, Cocoa or Cacao, Soy products	Artificial Fruit Juice, Colored Spirits and Liqueurs, Cider, Beers, White Wine, Sugary and Artificially Sweetened Drinks, Energy Drinks

Besides the Rare Adipose Disorder Diet, healthcare professionals also recommend some foods to, particularly, reduce inflammation. Strictly avoid genetically modified foods (GM foods) and factory-farmed meat. A list of such foods is mentioned below:

• Fruits and vegetables including apple, guava, strawberries, pumpkin, watermelon, plums, figs, peaches, broccoli, spinach, cabbage, mushrooms, asparagus, etc.
• Herbs and spices such as turmeric, cinnamon, ginger, mint, onions, cloves, oregano, thyme, and pepper
• Oils like flaxseed oil, olive oil, coconut oil, and sesame seed
• Some seafood such as trout, oysters, and tuna

LIPEDEMA DIET PLAN

T ake some time to understand what you are eating and what is in the food you are buying.

Below is a detailed description, explaining all the steps, from what food you should buy, how you have to choose the best foods, to how to use them on a daily basis. In this chapter, a 3-week plan is made for you people including a 7-day meal plan starting from week 2.

Make sure your diet is high in fiber; try to include a balance of foods including fish, pulses, nuts, and beans. Nuts like Brazil nuts and high in selenium nuts would help improve your metabolism.

Week 1: Prepare yourself

Gear yourself up for a positive start. Take a stance enthusiastically and with a determination that if you are diagnosed with lipedema, life doesn't end up here. You have to live a healthy and happy life for yourself.

In the previous chapter, you have read about the food that you have to remove from your diet and all those that you have to eat. So, in the beginning, just try to add valuable foods and try to avoid unwanted and harmful items.

Walk to a nearby store by yourself and shop for vegetables, fruits, olive oil, and other products taking help from table 1 (chapter 3). A very important thing while shopping for the best foods is reading and understanding food labeling. For example, if you are going to buy a bottle of extra virgin olive oil, below is a sample of extra virgin oil prepared in Morocco and approved by ONSSA (National Office for the Sanitary Protection of Food Products).

- ACIDITY: Must be ≤ 0.8%
- PEROXIDE: Must be ≤ 20 MEQ O2/kg
- WAX CONTENT: Must be≤ 250 MG/KG
- UV ABS K232: Must be ≤ 2.50
- K232: Must be ≤ 0.22

Here:
- ≤ shows that the given quantity should be equal or less than the mentioned percentage.
- UV ABS K232 and K232 can give us information about the quality and oxidative alteration

This is just a sample, consult a dietician and follow prescribed recommendations while reading the food labels.

If you love gardening, start growing seasonal vegetables on your own. This will also keep you active and mobile. And also add a precious hand-grown bulk of fresh veggies to your diet.

In the previous chapter, it has been explained in detail that processed food is a poison to all people facing Fat-related issues. These issues could be obesity, lymphedema, lipedema, etc. Processed foods lack natural minerals and nutrients. Start developing a habit of avoiding processed foods.

You can take a diary with you and write down what you felt while eating a portion of processed food and what you observed while leaving it.

Week 2: Add and Remove
As you know you make up your mind to fight lipedema. Keep on doing the activities of the first week and just add a little more to it.

During this week, get yourself prepared to follow a 7-day meal plan. You have to be strict in this regard because from week 3 you will have to follow a more uncompromising diet plan.

● Day 1 and 2:

Add egg, brown rice, or bread to your breakfast. Start eating fruit and go for vegetables cooked in suggested oils from Table 1. Keep yourself away from white rice and meat.

● Days 3 and 4:

Now start taking herbal teas (of your choice). Prefer to drink tea at night. Along with this remove artificial and processed fruit juices from your drink and try to have the fresh juice. Moreover, make a habit of walking before sleep and never lay down for rest just after eating, especially at night. Keep your dinner simple and oil-free.

● Day 5, 6, and 7:

If you are a sweet lover, then start practicing to minimize sugar in your diet. This is the most crucial stage no doubt. Yes, you can have brown sugar that should not be processed or refined.

During this week you can also practice simple and healthy cooking tips. The last chapter of this guide contains several healthy and easy-to-cook recipes. Make sure to take uncooked or half-cooked vegetables. Instead of frying, use boiling techniques for cooking. Adopt all such eating habits which keep you away from oils and fats.

Week 3: 7-day diet Plan

In the third week you have to follow a diet plan, which is obviously not rigid. You can alter and modify it according to your priorities and recommendations from a healthcare professional.

Days	Breakfast	Lunch	Dinner
1st	Egg, brown bread	Salmon salad with lettuce, cucumber, and tomato	Chickpeas, hummus with cauliflower rice

2nd	Whole grains, milk (sheep), Berries	Tuna with Beans, tomato, onion + oil (from table 1)	purple sprouting broccoli, and sweet potato mash o Herbal tea
3rd	Avocado, butter+ whole grains	Broccoli, quinoa and almonds,	Chicken and mushroom
4th	Home-Made Smoothies	Salmon salad with lettuce and corn	Vegetables, lentils, unsalted nuts
5th	Buckwheat with raspberries and cherries	Vegetable soup and brown rice	Recommended Seafood and avocados
6th	Egg, Apple slices	Minted pea and feta omelet	Cabbage, mushroom, Brazilian nuts
7th	Blueberries, oat bowl	Carrot orange and avocado salad	Salmon with sweet potato and corn salad

Start following this plan. You can change vegetables as per your choice. Don't forget to sprinkle herbs and spices on your meals including mint, coriander, cinnamon, turmeric, pepper, oregano, thyme, etc. if you feel hungry some other time other than breakfast, lunch, and dinner, take fruits and nuts as snacks.

Make a routine of taking any herbal tea before bed.

Remain stick to the diet plan, created for you in Table 2. Follow the plan and write down the consequences in it. What do you feel after eating specific foods? Do you notice a reduction in swelling and inflammation? If yes, then well and good. If not, opt for other combinations of food for your meals and observe.

Now you are trained enough to follow the diet plan. Must consult your healthcare professional and do follow his/her prescriptions as well including medication and maybe liposuction, if recommended.

SAMPLE RECIPES

Garlic Hummus

Ingredients:
- 12 heads of garlic, roasted
- 2 tsp. virgin coconut oil
- 2 12-cup muffin tins
- extra trays of ice cube

Instructions:
1. Preheat the oven to 400°F.
2. Cut off the top of each garlic head to make the top of the cloves visible.
3. Put each garlic head in a muffin tin cup.
4. Rub the top of garlic heads with coconut oil.
5. Use the second muffin tin to cover the first one.
6. Put in the oven and wait for 30 minutes to bake.
7. Take the garlic cloves out of the heads.
8. You may place 4-5 cloves of garlic in each ice cube tray section to store leftovers.
9. Use olive oil to cover cloves and freeze.
10. Squeeze the frozen roasted garlic cubes out of the trays and store them using a container.

Salmon and Asparagus

Ingredients:
- 2 salmon filets
- 14-oz. young potatoes
- 8 asparagus spears, trimmed and halved
- 2 handfuls cherry tomatoes
- 1 handful basil leaves
- 2 tbsp. extra-virgin olive oil
- 1 tbsp. balsamic vinegar

Instructions:
1. Heat oven to 428°F.
2. Arrange potatoes into a baking dish.
3. Drizzle potatoes with extra-virgin olive oil.
4. Roast potatoes until they have turned golden brown.
5. Place asparagus into the baking dish together with the potatoes.
6. Roast in the oven for 15 minutes.
7. Arrange cherry tomatoes and salmon among the vegetables.
8. Drizzle with balsamic vinegar and the remaining olive oil.
9. Roast until the salmon is cooked.
10. Throw in basil leaves before transferring everything to a serving dish.
11. Serve while hot.

Tahini Salmon

Instructions:
- 1/4 cup tahini
- 3 tbsp. fresh lemon juice
- 1 tsp. mashed garlic
- 1/4 tsp. salt
- 1/2 cup finely chopped cilantro
- 2 tbsp. roughly chopped toasted walnuts
- 2 tbsp. roughly chopped toasted almonds
- 1 tbsp. finely chopped onion
- 1 tsp. extra-virgin olive oil
- cayenne
- black pepper, freshly ground
- 1 lb. wild salmon skin removed, fresh or frozen

Instructions:
1. In a bowl, combine the tahini, 2 tbsp. of lemon juice, 3 tbsp. of water, mashed garlic, and 1/8 tsp. of salt; set aside
2. In a separate bowl, combine the cilantro, walnuts, almonds, onion, olive oil, cayenne, black pepper, and 1/8 tsp. of salt.
3. Fill the bottom of a steamer with water and bring to a boil.
4. Season fish with 1 tbsp. of lemon juice.
5. Place it on a plate and put it on the top of the steamer. Cover and cook, taking care to remove while the fish is still pink inside, about 3 to 4 minutes.
6. Remove the fish from the steamer, top with the tahini mixture, and then with the cilantro mixture.
7. Serve warm or at room temperature.

Salmon with Avocados and Brussels Sprout

Ingredients:
- 2 lbs. of salmon filet, divided into 4 pieces
- 1 tsp. ground cumin
- 1 tsp. onion powder
- 1 tsp. paprika powder
- 1/2 tsp. garlic powder
- 1 tsp. chili powder
- Himalayan sea salt
- black pepper, freshly grounded

Avocado sauce:
- 2 chopped avocados
- 1 lime, squeezed for the juice
- 1 tbsp. extra-virgin olive oil
- 1 tbsp. fresh minced cilantro
- 1 diced small red onion
- 1 minced garlic clove
- Himalayan sea salt to taste
- black pepper, freshly grounded

Brussels sprout:
- 3 lbs. of Brussels Sprout
- 1/2 cup raw honey
- 1/2 cup balsamic vinegar
- 1/2 cup melted coconut oil
- 1 cup dried cranberries
- Himalayan sea salt
- black pepper, freshly grounded

Instructions:
To make the salmon and avocado sauce:
1. Combine cumin, onion, chili powder, garlic, and paprika seasoned with salt and pepper. Mix well before dry rubbing on the salmon.
2. Place the salmon in the fridge for 30 minutes.

3. Preheat the grill.

4. In a bowl, mash avocado until texture becomes smooth. Pour in all the remaining ingredients and mix thoroughly.

5. Grill salmon for 5 minutes on each side or until cooked.

6. Drizzle avocado on cooked salmon.

To make the Brussel Sprout:

1. Preheat the oven to 375°F.

2. Mix Brussels Sprout with coconut oil. Season with salt and pepper.

3. Place vegetables on a baking sheet and roast for about 30 minutes.

4. In a separate pan, combine vinegar and honey.

5. Simmer in slow heat until it boils and thickens.

6. Drizzle them on top of the Brussels Sprouts.

7. Serve with the salmon.

Chicken Breast Delight

Ingredients:
- 1 tsp. dried oregano
- 1/2 tsp. rosemary
- 1/2 tsp. garlic powder
- 1/8 tsp. salt
- finely ground black pepper
- 4 chicken breasts

Instructions:
1. Remove any fat from the breasts.
2. Mix the remaining ingredients in a separate container.
3. Add the mixture on either side of the chicken.
4. Prepare a frying pan, lightly oil the pan, and set the stove to medium.
5. Add the chicken into the frying pan. Cook for 3 to 5 minutes on each face.
6. Cool the chicken for a couple of minutes after cooking.
7. Serve warm.

Garlic Broccoli Salad

Ingredients:
- 1 head broccoli, cut into florets
- 1 tsp. olive oil
- 1-1/2 tbsp. rice wine vinegar
- 1 tbsp. sesame oil
- 2 cloves garlic, minced
- 1 pinch cayenne pepper
- 3 tbsp. golden raisins

Instructions:
1. Fill water into a steamer. Bring to a boil.
2. Add broccoli. Cover. Steam until tender for about 3 minutes.
3. Rinse broccoli and set aside.
4. Heat olive oil in a skillet over medium heat.
5. Put in pine nuts. Stir fry for 1-2 minutes.
6. Remove from heat.
7. Whisk together rice vinegar, sesame oil, pepper, and garlic.
8. Transfer the broccoli, nuts, and raisins to the rice vinegar dressing.
9. Serve and enjoy.

Mixed Vegetable Roast with Lemon Zest

Ingredients:
- 1-1/2 cups broccoli florets
- 1-1/2 cups cauliflower florets
- 3/4 cup red bell pepper, diced
- 3/4 cup zucchini, diced
- 2 thinly sliced cloves of garlic
- 2 tsp. lemon zest
- 1 tbsp. olive oil
- a pinch of salt
- 1 tsp. dried and crushed oregano

Instructions:
1. Preheat the oven at 425°F for 25 minutes.
2. Combine garlic and florets of broccoli and cauliflower in a baking pan.
3. Drizzle oil evenly over the vegetables. Season with salt and oregano.
4. Stir the vegetables to coat them evenly.
5. Place the pan inside the oven and roast for 10 minutes.
6. Add zucchini and bell pepper to the mix. Toss to combine.
7. Continue roasting for 10 to 15 minutes more until the vegetables turn light brown.
8. Drizzle lemon zest over vegetables and toss.
9. Serve and enjoy.

Baked Salmon

Ingredients:
- 2 salmon fillets
- 6 cups of fresh spinach
- 2 tsp. coconut oil
- 1/4 tsp. garlic powder
- 1/4 tsp. turmeric
- 3 large cloves of garlic
- lemon juice
- salt
- pepper

Instructions:
1. Preheat the oven to 400°F.
2. Line a baking dish with parchment paper.
3. Marinate salmon fillets in lemon juice, coconut oil, garlic powder, turmeric, salt, and pepper.
4. Let it sit for a few minutes. This may also be done the night before to help the juices and flavor get into the salmon.
5. Once the oven is ready, bake salmon for 15 minutes.
6. Cook some of the garlic in a pan with coconut oil.
7. Add spinach and cook until ready. Season with salt and pepper to taste.
8. Take salmon out of the oven and put spinach beside it.
9. Serve and enjoy.

Roasted Chicken

Ingredients:
- 1 whole organic chicken
- 2 sprigs organic rosemary
- 2 garlic cloves
- 1 tbsp. herbes de Provence
- 1 tbsp. coarse sea salt

Instructions:
1. Preheat the oven to 350°F.
2. Put the chicken on a baking pan or glass Pyrex, breast facing up.
3. Stuff the cavity with the rosemary and garlic cloves.
4. Sprinkle half of the salt and herbes de Provence on the breast. Turn the chicken breast side down. Sprinkle the remaining salt and herb mix on the top.
5. Bake for about 1-1/2 hours. The skin should be nicely browned when the chicken is ready.
6. Serve immediately with a salad, or side dish of choice, drizzling on the cooking fat from the roasting pan.

Spinach and Watercress Salad

Ingredients:
- 1 cup watercress, washed with stems removed
- 3 cups baby spinach, washed with stems removed
- 1 medium sliced avocado
- 1/4 cup avocado oil
- 1/8 cup lemon juice
- a pinch of salt

Instructions:
1. Pat dry the spinach and watercress. Remove the stem and separate the leaves.
2. On a large serving plate, combine the leaves of the watercress and the spinach.
3. Cut the avocado in half, then remove the pit. Peel the skin off from each side.
4. Slice the avocados into thin strips. Set aside.
5. Prepare the dressing by combining avocado oil and lemon juice.
6. Arrange the avocado strips on top of the watercress and spinach.
7. Season with salt and pepper.

Vegetable Broth

Ingredients:
- 1 tbsp. oil
- 2 leeks, sliced
- 2 carrots, sliced
- 2 ribs celery
- 1/4 tsp. salt
- 8 cups water

To make the soup:
- 1 tbsp. oil
- 2 cups potatoes, diced
- 1 cup mushrooms, diced
- 1-1/2 cups cauliflower, diced
- 1 cup onion, diced
- 1 cup celery, diced
- 1 cup carrot, diced
- 1-1/2 cups red beans, cooked
- 2 sprigs rosemary
- 4 sprigs thyme
- 2 cups spinach

Instructions:
1. To a pot on medium heat, add oil and leeks.
2. Cook for about three minutes or until they start to soften up.
3. Add carrots and top of a few celery stalks with leaves.
4. Cover with water.
5. Add salt. Bring to a simmer and cook until carrots are very tender but not mushy.
6. Turn off the heat and let it cool down a little.
7. When the broth has cooled down, strain out the veggies.
8. Remove carrots and set them aside.
9. Squeeze most of the liquid out of the leeks and celery.

To cook the soup:
1. Add carrots to some of the broth and blend.

2. With a pot on medium heat, add oil, onions, raw carrots, and celery. Cook until onions are translucent, approximately 3 to 5 minutes.

3. Add broth, potatoes, and herbs.

4. Bring to a simmer and cook for 10 minutes.

5. Add cauliflower and red beans.

6. Simmer for another 5 minutes.

7. Add the package of frozen green beans and cook until the potatoes and cauliflower are tender, approximately for another 5 minutes.

8. At the end of cooking, add spinach.

9. Serve warm.

Salad Medley

Ingredients:
- 4 artichokes, halved
- 1/2 avocado, sliced into thin wedges
- 1/2 red, yellow, or green bell pepper, thinly sliced
- 1/4 squash, thinly sliced
- 1/2 zucchini, thinly sliced
- 1/2 red, yellow, or green onion, thinly sliced
- 1 cup mushrooms, thinly sliced
- 1 cup broccoli
- 1/4 cup broccoli sprouts
- 1 cup cauliflower
- 1 cup spinach
- 1 cup kale
- 1 bunch leeks, chopped
- 1/4 cup raw sunflower seeds, sprouted
- 1/4 cup raw almonds, sprouted
- 1/4 cup garbanzo beans, sprouted
- 1/4 cup mung beans, sprouted
- 1/4 cup red or green lentils, sprouted
- 1/4 cup purple cabbage, shredded
- 2 tbsp. extra-virgin olive oil

Instructions:
1. Steam vegetables in a saucepan with 1-inch water for 5 to 10 minutes.
2. Transfer steamed vegetables into a serving bowl.
3. Drizzle with extra-virgin olive oil.
4. Toss the vegetables.
5. Serve immediately.

Quinoa Lentil Salad

Ingredients:
- 2/3 cups dried brown lentils
- 2 cups water
- 1 cup quinoa
- 1 yellow sweet peppers, diced
- 1 shallot, chopped
- 1 bunch arugula, finely chopped
- 2 tsp. Dijon mustard
- 1/4 cup lemon juice
- 1/4 cup extra virgin olive oil
- 1/3 cup crumbled feta cheese
- 1 pinch salt
- 4 tbsp. fresh mint, chopped

Instructions:
1. Bring 2 cups of saltwater to a boil in a saucepan.
2. Toss veggies into boiling saltwater. Lower heat, and cook for 30 minutes.
3. Drain lentils and discard water. Set veggies aside.
4. Boil another batch of saltwater, and cook the quinoa in the pan.
5. In a bowl, mix pepper, salt, mustard, lemon juice, and oil.
6. Place veggies in a larger bowl, and pour the mixture.
7. Sprinkle mint and feta cheese over the salad.
8. Serve and enjoy

Fruit and Dark Greens Salad

Ingredients:
- 1 cup watermelon
- 1 cup cucumber sliced or spiral
- 1/2 cup raspberries
- 1 sliced avocado
- 1 cup baby broccoli
- 1 cup papaya
- 1/2 cup toasted almonds
- 4 cups baby kale

Dressing:
- 1/2 cup olive oil
- 1/2 cup master tonic
- 1/4 cup goji berries
- 4 dates
- a pinch of sea salt

Tonic:
- 1/4 cup garlic, minced
- 1/4 cup onion, chopped
- 2 tbsp. horseradish, minced
- 2 knobs turmeric, chopped
- 1 jalapeno pepper, chopped
- 32 oz. organic apple cider vinegar
- 1/4 cup fresh ginger, chopped
- juice of 1 lemon

Instructions:
1. Mix all salad ingredients except almonds.
2. Toss salad.

To make the dressing:
1. Mix master tonic, olive oil, and salt together.
2. In a blender, blend goji berries and dates until smooth.

3. Upon serving the salad, drizzle the dressing on, and gently add almonds.

To make the master tonic:
1. Add all ingredients to apple cider vinegar.
2. Blend all ingredients until everything is mixed well.
3. Let tonic sit in a jar for 1 to 2 weeks, shaking periodically.
4. Strain first before adding the leftover vinegar mixture into a jar with a cover.

CONCLUSION

As shown, lipedema is a commonly spread disorder mostly targeting women. Serious action is needed for its correct diagnosis and awareness about its differentiation from obesity.

Although specific diet and addition and removal of food items from the diet cannot guarantee a cure, following a healthy diet plan could help one manage lipedema.

This guide has outlined various foods to avoid and to include as well as a sample 3-week plan to implement.

If you have enjoyed this guide, please leave a review. Thank you again and good luck on your journey to better health.

REFERENCES

7 recommended foods for lipedema. (2021, September 28). Lipepedia. https://lipepedia.com/en/7-recommended-foods-for-lipedema/.

Buck, Donald W, and Karen L Herbst. "Lipedema: A Relatively Common Disease with Extremely Common Misconceptions." Plastic and reconstructive surgery. Global open. Wolters Kluwer Health, September 28, 2016. https://www.ncbi.nlm.nih.gov/pmc/articles/PMC5055019/.

FRACS, D. N. S. M., PhD. (n.d.). What to eat to manage lipoedema. Retrieved August 26, 2022, from https://www.naveensomia.com.au/myblog/what-to-eat-to-manage-lipoedema.

Lipedema Foundation. Accessed February 8, 2022. https://www.lipedema.org/.

Lipedema of the Legs; a Syndrome Characterized by Fat Legs and Edema. Annals of internal medicine. U.S. National Library of Medicine. Accessed February 8, 2022. https://pubmed.ncbi.nlm.nih.gov/14830102/.

Lipedema: A Giving Smarter Guide - Milken Institute. Accessed February 8, 2022. https://milkeninstitute.org/sites/default/files/reports-pdf/Lipedema-Giving-Smarter-Guide.pdf.

Lipedema: Symptoms, causes, tests and treatment. (n.d.). Cleveland Clinic. Retrieved August 26, 2022, from https://my.clevelandclinic.org/health/diseases/17175-lipedema.

Lipoedema—Better health channel. (n.d.). Retrieved August 26, 2022, from https://www.betterhealth.vic.gov.au/health/conditionsandtreatments/Lipoedema.

Nutrition. (n.d.). Lipedema.Com. Retrieved August 26, 2022, from https://www.lipedema.com/self-care/nutrition.

Rad Diet. Cure Lipedema. Accessed February 8, 2022. http://www.curelipedema.org/rad-diet.

Shin, B. W., Sim, Y.-J., Jeong, H. J., & Kim, G. C. (2011). Lipedema, a rare disease. Annals of Rehabilitation Medicine, 35(6), 922–927. https://doi.org/10.5535/arm.2011.35.6.922.

The Rad Diet. Welcome. Accessed February 8, 2022. https://lipedemanetworkcanada.com/the-rad-diet/.

Treating Lipedema. Lipedema Foundation. Accessed February 8, 2022. https://www.lipedema.org/treating-lipedema.

What Women Should Know about Lipedema. Cleveland Clinic, October 5, 2021. https://health.clevelandclinic.org/heres-what-you-should-know-about-lipedema-a-condition-that-causes-excess-fat-in-the-legs/.

Women's Experiences of Living with Lipedema. Taylor & Francis. Accessed February 8, 2022. https://www.tandfonline.com/doi/full/10.1080/07399332.2021.1932894.